Diabetes

Step by Step Diet Guide on Delicious and Healthy Foods You can Eat

Hello, Stevie Anderson here. Thank you for purchasing my book. As a gift to you from me, I am allowing you to enter into my V.I.P. list. I am only allowing a certain amount of people in my V.I.P. list. Once it's filled up, it's closed forever. Inside my V.I.P. list you will get the priceless opportunity to get my new books on personal development absolutely FREE when it is released.

To find out more about my V.I.P list Click Here

or go to http://tokkul.com/personal-development

This is a limited time offer to join in the V.I.P group.

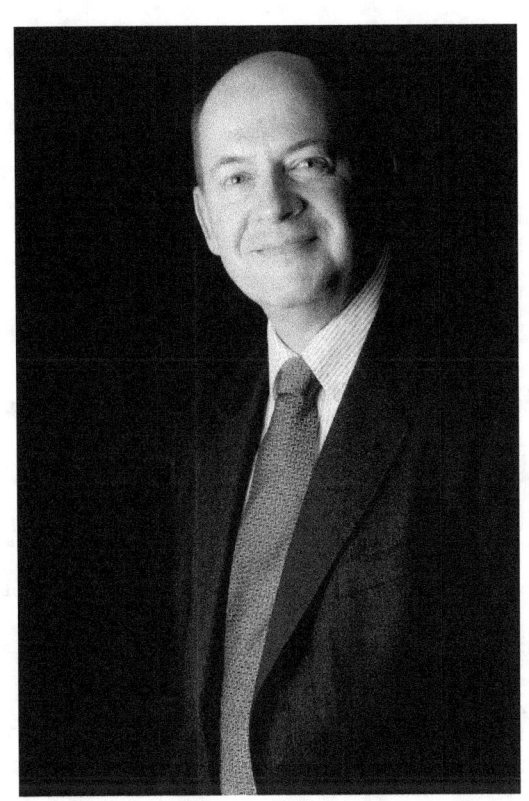

Contents

Lunch is the best time for diabetics to really enjoy their food. You will find some very simple recipes that will help you have an idea of what a low fat, low carb tasty meal should really look like.

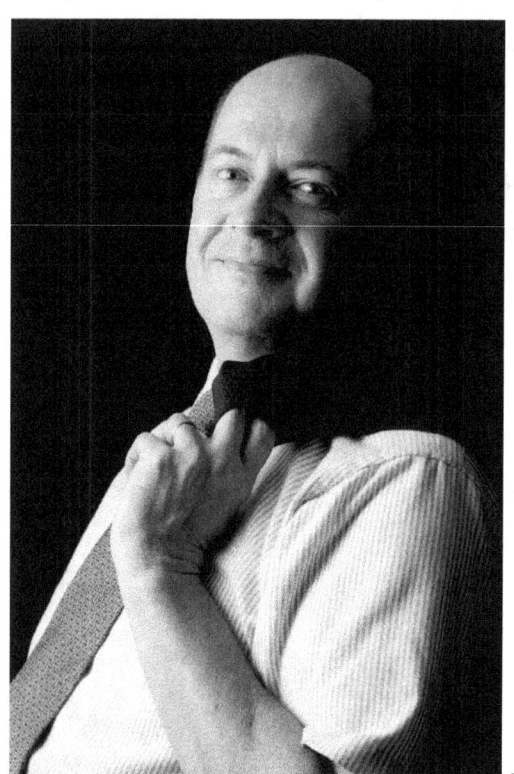

Introduction

I want to thank you and congratulate you for downloading the book, *"Diabetes: Step by Step Diet Guide on Delicious and Healthy Foods You Can Eat"*.

This book contains proven steps and strategies on how to actually prepare delicious meals for people who suffer from Diabetes. After carefully observing and doing my own research I've realized that diabetics often felt condemned to eat the same menus or restrict themselves from eating certain foods because they simply feared that these meals might have too much salt or too much sugar. So, most of the time, they will stick to eating boiled vegetables or boiled meat for lunch or dinner. Another thing that really attracted my attention were the data provided by the American Diabetes Association, which stipulates that over 29.1 million Americans are affected by the disease. This means that many of them may not always feel enthusiastic enough to try something better (that is still right for them), because, let's face it; it is a complicated disease to cope with.

I want people who suffer from the condition and who love to cook (or anyone who is interested in cooking for a diabetic person) to have more than the sometimes monotonous meals, which are most of the time watery and over boiled with no taste at all.

Cooking tastier meals as a diabetic or for a diabetic person should make eating a celebration rather than a simple routine. You should want to wake up and eat something that you enjoy eating or again go to bed with the idea that the next day, you will wake up to have the meal of your life.

Let us now discover a new and brighter side of being diabetic, which is to eat what you can enjoy. But first, let me give you a brief reminder of what Diabetes is.

Thanks again for downloading this book, I hope you enjoy it!

Chapter 1: Important Facts About Diabetes

What do Diabetics Normally eat?

This is an essential question, for people who cater for diabetic people, but also for people who have perhaps, recently been diagnosed with the disease. If you are not a great cook or are a bit paranoid because of the stress this disease puts on you, you don't have to worry; this guide will provide you with just enough information you'll need to prepare better meals.

As you certainly know it, diabetes is a metabolic disease in which the body is unable to produce any (or low levels) of insulin, which in turn, leads to high levels of glucose in the blood. This means that if you (or someone you know) doesn't control the disease by restricting his or her intake of sugar or salt he or she will develop retinopathy (or disease of the eye), nephropathy (disease of the kidneys) and neuropathy (disease of the nerves), in the long run.

So, this disease basically requires sufferers to have a strict diet. The appropriate type of food should be low in glycemic index (or GI). Low glycemic food normally has an index equal to 55 or less. So foods like white bread, for instance, which have a glycemic index of 100 are to be avoided. Whether you are a Type 2, type 1, affected by prediabetes or gestational diabetes (which affects some pregnant women), you would have to eat food that can provide enough Calcium, fiber, magnesium, vitamin A, C and E to your body.

In conclusion, diabetics need more or less the same nutrients as "ordinary" people, but they just have to eat moderate portions of these foods, compared to them.

Calorie Count Per Day

According to the American Diabetes Association, the number of calories needed by a diabetic person depends on gender, size, weight, age, height, how active this person is and also on whether the person is pregnant or not.

Another thing that is important to note is that although a person who is active (which means that this person works out regularly additionally to her or his regular activities) requires a greater amount of calorie intake. This need tends to decrease as the person ages. For instance, a sedentary 18-year-old male will need a daily intake of 2400 calories while a more active person in the same age range will need an intake of 3200 calories.

 Now, a diabetic person who is 76-year-old will need 2000 calories if he is not active and 2400 calories if he has a very active lifestyle. On another part, it also appears that women tend to need less caloric intake than men, where for instance, a non-active 18-year-old woman would need 1800 calories and a very active one would need 2400 calories. As women with diabetes, get older, they too seem to require less calorie intake, since a 76-year-old women would need 1600 calories if she's not active and 400 more calories (2000 calories) when she is active. These are some of the major points to keep in mind when cooking for a diabetic person (whether it's you or someone else).

What is The "Right Food" Doing to Their System?

The types of food that will be used in our guide, bring an enormous number of benefits to diabetics. Some, like dark chocolate, will reduce insulin resistance, improve insulin sensitivity, drop insulin levels and will stop blunt cravings. Oily fish like salmon and raw vegetables like broccoli have anti-inflammatory benefits and can even improve blood sugar control and protect blood vessels. And fruits like berries helps flush fat out of the system. All of these ingredients are regularly used to make delicious dishes for diabetics.

How Many Times a Day do They Normally Eat?

For those of you who can remember, 30 years or 20 years ago, diabetic people were restrained to a very strict diet, where they had to respect every recommendation given by their health specialist.

Now, things are more flexible and we can thank scientific research for that. Diabetic people have, in fact, more freedom to choose what they put on their plate, but they still have to control their intake of carbohydrates, to limit high rates of blood glucose.

The very firm recommendation, when organizing your meals as a diabetic, is to try to eat the same amount of carbohydrates for every meal and to never skip breakfast (because it helps jump start your metabolism). Also, for those who are active (workout a lot) or take fix doses of medication, it is recommended to take a snack or two, during the day.

What Should You Always Put in Your Shopping List?

Make sure you pack up in foods that are low on the Glycemic index (or GI). I've set up a list of foods that are not only delicious, but that will also provide key nutrients such as Calcium, Potassium, Fiber, Magnesium, vitamins (A, C, and E) and most of all, are safe to eat for diabetic people.

-Beans: They are high in fiber and with just half a cup you can get 1/3 of your daily requirement in magnesium and potassium. You can use canned beans, but make sure it is drained and rinsed off to get rid of the sodium and other preservatives.

-Dark green leafy vegetables: Like spinach, collards and kale. They are low in calories and carbohydrates but, they should be eaten in moderation.

-Citrus fruits: Like Grapefruit, oranges, lemons and limes. These are considered to be rich in soluble fibers and vitamin C.

-Sweet potatoes: They are full of vitamin A and fibers.

-Berries: Like blueberries and strawberries. They are packed with antioxidants; vitamins and fiber.

-Tomatoes: They are rich in vitamin C, Iron and Vitamin E.

-Fish high in Omega-3 fatty acids like Salmon.

-Whole grains: They are rich in magnesium, chromium, and folate.

-Nuts: They are rich in magnesium and fiber.

-Fat-free milk and yogurt: They will provide you with your necessary intake of Calcium and vitamin D.

You have the option to buy them fresh, frozen or canned (especially fish and vegetables).

This is an attempt to give an idea of how you can organize your pantry or refrigerator, with diabetic super foods like these ones. Make sure you always have them, because you will use a lot of it for flavor and their nutritional value.

Let us now move on to our first ideas for delicious meals that should be suitable for diabetics.

Chapter 2: Original Breakfast Ideas

Breakfast is supposed to be the actual meal that jump starts you for the rest of the day. What is better to do than cook one that has just enough nutrition for the day, but that you also enjoy eating?

Most of us, I suppose don't like to eat in the morning, but if you suffer from type 2 diabetes, for instance, you have no other options but to eat in the morning, otherwise your body will weaken considerably during the day.

You have the choice between a light breakfast for people who don't like eating too much in the morning but still can gain the essential nutrients for the day and breakfast options for the diabetics who work out in the morning and definitely need to eat something consistent.

Note that to evaluate the consistency of each meal, the amount of calories and carbohydrates per serving is used. This is to help you quickly identify not only the amount of fat and sugar found in one serving but also evaluate the nutritional value it has.

Let's begin with something light for the not so hungry.

A Simple Breakfast Plan for The Not So Hungry

Breakfast Number One: The Breakfast Shake (104 cal. and 20g of carb per serving)

For four servings you will need:

- Some fat-free milk or if you prefer some plain nonfat yogurt

- ½ cup of fruits (you have the choice between strawberries, bananas, and blueberries).

- 1 teaspoon of wheat germ.

- 1 teaspoon of nut

- Some ice.

Directions:

Blend your ingredients together. Make sure it's perfectly liquefied and drink right away to take advantage of the nutritional benefits. To make things even faster you can prepare your fruits (diced or chopped) the night before.

Breakfast Number Two: Tasty Bran Muffins (200 cal. and 20g carb per serving)

For 12 muffins you will need:

- 1 cup of whole wheat flour.

- 1 teaspoon of baking powder

- 1.2 teaspoon of salt

- 1 cup of natural bran

- 1 cup of buttermilk or 1 cup of sour milk.

- 1/3 cup of cooking oil

- ¼ cup of unsweetened apple sauce.

- 1 egg

- ¼ cup of Splenda granular

- ½ teaspoon of vanilla

- 1 cup of berries

Directions:

Use a large bowl to mix the flour, baking powder, and soda, the salt, and butter. In another bowl, mix the buttermilk with the bran and let it stand for 5 minutes. Next, add the rest of the ingredients to the bran mixture. Fill your greased muffin cups (3/4 full). Bake your muffins at 375 degrees for about 20 to 25 minutes. Remove your muffins from the oven and let it stand for 5 minutes. Then, remove them from the pan.

To make it even tastier, top your muffins with a dollop of low or nonfat yogurt and enjoy!

Breakfast Number Three: Breakfast burrito (200 cal. and 15g of carb per serving)

You will need:

- 4 eggs.

- 4 egg whites

- Dash hot pepper sauce

- 2 tablespoons of reduced fat cheddar cheese (preferably shredded).

- ¼ teaspoons of ground black pepper.

- 2 teaspoons of trans fat-free margarine.

- ¼ cup of diced onions

- 4 slices of reduced sodium deli style ham (about 3 ounces).

- ¼ cup of diced green pepper.

- 4 heated corn tortillas.

- 4 teaspoons of salsa.

Directions:

Use a medium sized bowl for your preparation. Mix the eggs, egg whites, hot pepper sauce, the black pepper and the cheese. Melt the margarine in a medium non-stick pan, over medium heat. Place the ham in the pan and sauté for 3 minutes, then remove it from the pan. Reduce your cooking heat to low and add the eggs to the pan. Stir the eggs with a spatula until the eggs are cooked. Divide the egg mixture evenly into 4 servings. Put each portion of the mixture into a tortilla and top each one of them with one teaspoon of salsa, then, fold the tortilla to close.

Breakfast Number Four: Almonds and Fruits (less than 300 calories)

Simply eat a handful of whole raw almonds added to a small serving of fruits such as peach, berries, orange or apple (pick one of them). This simple and fast breakfast, rich in fiber and monounsaturated fats (in the almonds) will fill you up. The fruits will add a touch of sweetness to it.

A Few Tips That Can Help Simplify Your Cooking:

When cooking, use less fat by using nonstick pans and cooking sprays or heart healthy butter substitutes.

Avoid fat and sugar-laden coffee drinks. Instead, drink regular coffee with some 2% low-fat milk and sugar substitutes.

Complex Breakfast Menus

As we said earlier, eating right and at the right time is necessary for diabetics. If you like working out in the morning, or just love to have a consistent breakfast when you wake up, then you might want to try one of these delicious recipes...

Complex Breakfast Number One: Pear-Ginger Pancakes (242 cal. and 39-gram carbs)

For 4 servings, you will need:

- ½ cup of all-purpose flour.

- ½ cup of whole wheat flour.

- 2 teaspoons of baking powder

- 1 tablespoon of brown sugar or brown sugar substitute.

- 1/8 teaspoon of salt

- ¼ teaspoon of ground ginger

- ¾ cup of fat-free milk

- ¼ cup of refrigerated (or frozen) egg product, thawed or 1 egg

- 2 tablespoons of canola oil

- ½ of a medium pear, cored and finely chopped (1/2 cup)

- And apricot syrup (that you will prepare yourself, as well).

Direction:

Use a medium bowl to mix your all-purpose flour with the whole wheat flour, the brown sugar, baking powder, the ginger, and salt. Then, make a well in the center of the mixture. In a separate and smaller bowl, whisk together the egg, milk and oil and stir it in your chopped pear. Add the egg mixture to the flour mixture previously made and stir until everything is moistened. Then, pour ¼ cup of the mixture into a hot greased pan. Make sure you spread the batter evenly in your pan. Cook each pancake on medium heat for a maximum of 4 minutes. When done, you can serve with warm apricot-pear syrup.

*To make the apricot syrup you will need (for ½ a cup): ½ of a medium pear (finely chopped and cored), 1 tablespoon of lemon juice, 2 tablespoons of low sugar apricot preserves, 1 tablespoon of water, and 1/8 teaspoon of ground ginger.

Directions: Use a small saucepan where you will combine your chopped pear and the lemon juice. Mix in the preserves, the water and your ginger. Melt the preserves on low heat with your mixture. Stir occasionally until all is melted and warm. When ready, pour it on top of your pancakes.

Useful tip: To keep your pancakes warm while you make the syrup, you can keep them in a 300-degree F hot oven.

Complex Breakfast Number Two: Scrambled Eggs with sausage (198 cal. and 32-gram carbs).

For 2 servings you will need:

- 2 eggs

- 2 tablespoons of reduced sodium chicken broth

- An ounce of sliced cooked turkey sausage

- ¼ cup of quartered cherry tomatoes

- Pinch ground pepper

- 2 tablespoons of finely shredded reduced fat cheddar cheese

- 1 whole grain English muffin, which should be halved and toasted

Directions:

Coat your pan with cooking spray and preheat it over medium heat. In a medium bowl, whisk together your eggs, broth, black pepper and stir in the sliced sausage. Pour the egg mixture into the hot pan and cook it on medium heat without stirring. Cook it until the mixture begins to set on the bottom and around the edges. With the help of a spatula lift and fold the half cooked egg mixture. Continue cooking over medium heat and add the tomatoes and cheese. Cook for about 1 minute more until the egg is fully cooked (make sure that it's still glossy and moist). Serve the egg over toasted English muffin halves.

Complex Breakfast Number Three: Cornmeal Waffles with Blueberry Compote (204 cal., 31 carb grams)

What you will need for 8 servings:

- ¾ cup of flour

- ½ cup of cornmeal

- 1 teaspoon of baking powder

- 2 tablespoons of packed brown sugar

- ¼ teaspoon of salt

- 1 cup of buttermilk

- 3 tablespoons of canola oil

- ½ cup of fat-free milk

- 2 egg yolks

- ½ teaspoon of vanilla

- 2 egg whites

Direction:

Use a large bowl to combine the flour, brown sugar, baking powder, and salt. In a separate medium size bowl, mix the buttermilk, milk, oil, egg yolks and vanilla together. Whisk the mixture (but not too much) and then whisk it into the flour mixture. Beat your egg whites in a big bowl until soft peaks form (you can use an electric mixer to do that). Fold your egg whites, gently into the batter.

For the Blueberry compote, you will need 1 cup of apple juice, 1 tablespoon of lemon juice, 2 cups of fresh blueberries, ½ teaspoon of finely shredded lemon peel, and 1/8 teaspoon of ground cinnamon.

Direction: In a medium saucepan, bring your apple juice and lemon juice to boiling and reduce the heat. Let it simmer for 8 to 10 minutes (until reduced by half, with the pan uncovered). Stir in the fresh blueberries, lemon peel and cinnamon. Return to boiling, reduce the heat. Let it simmer (uncovered) for 5 minutes. Pour the mixture on top of your waffles and enjoy.

Complex Breakfast Number Four: Asparagus-cheese Omelet (116 cal., 4 g carbs)

For 1 serving you will need:

- 3-5 thin spears asparagus

- 3 egg whites and 1 whole egg

- 1/8 teaspoon of freshly ground black pepper

- ½ teaspoon of olive oil

- An ounce of wrapped spreadable cut up cheese wedge of your choice

- 1 tablespoon of red sweet pepper slivers

- 1 teaspoon of fresh parsley or basil

Directions:

Spray your cooking spray all over your pan. Then, add your asparagus to the pan and pan roast it over medium-high heat for about 7 minutes. They should end up being crisp-tender, make sure you turn them occasionally. When done, set your asparagus aside. Use a medium bowl to mix your egg whites and pepper. Beat your egg whites with a fork until they are combined (but not frothy). Heat your oil over medium high heat, then, add your egg whites to your pan. After reducing the heat to medium, use a spatula to gently lift the edges of the set egg white (the liquid white egg should set under the set egg at this stage, so tilt your pan). Cook your egg until it's set but still moist. Arrange your asparagus in half of the eggs, in the pan. Top it with cheese. Fold the unfilled half of the eggs over the asparagus and cheese. Gently put your omelet on a serving plate. To finish, sprinkle your omelet with some red sweet pepper and parsley.

Chapter 3: Colorful and Delicious Snacks

Snacks are important for people with diabetes. They help them regain their energy during the day, especially when they are taking some medication to help with their condition. You will find in this chapter, a list of delicious snacks that you can enjoy all day long, without worrying about your sugar levels ever going up.

Your Midday Snacks

Green Papaya Salad (112 cal. and 18-gram carbs per serving)

What you will need for ¾ cup serving:

- 2 medium green (unripe) papayas

- 6 garlic cloves

- 6 small and stemmed Thai chili peppers

- Some stevia or Splenda for taste

- 3 tablespoons of fish sauce

- 1/2 cup of green beans, trimmed and cut into 2 inches' lengths

- 6 quartered cherry tomatoes

- 1/4 cup of roasted unsalted peanuts

- 1/4 cup of fresh lime juice

- 1 head Red leaf lettuce with leaves removed and washed

Directions:

First, Peel and cut in half (lengthwise) and seed the papayas. Cut them into long, thin shreds or have them shredded and set aside. Use a large mortar to combine the garlic and chilies and pound them into bits with a pestle. Then, add the sweetener and fish sauce and mix with the pestle. Add the papaya and green beans and pound for about 3 minutes to crush them (slightly). Use a spoon to scrape the sides (you should rotate the spoon around the mortar to do so). Then, add the cherry tomatoes and pound, once more, for about one minute to release some of their juices. Stir the mixture in the peanuts and lime juice. Place a few leaves of lettuce on each plate, spoon the salad onto the lettuce and enjoy!

Low Carb Cream Cheese muffins (127 cal.,49-gram carbs for one muffin):

You will need:

- 8oz. of cream cheese
- 2 large eggs
- 1/4 cup of Xylitol (natural sweetener)
- 1teaspoon of pure vanilla extract
- 3 tablespoons of vanilla whey protein
- ½ tablespoon of cinnamon
- ¼ teaspoon of pumpkin spice
- ¼ teaspoon of nutmeg

Directions:

Preheat the oven to 350 degrees. Mix all the ingredients together in a medium bowl. With an electric mixer, beat the ingredients until you have the consistency of a pancake batter. Spray your muffin tin with cooking spray and pour about 1/4 cup of batter into each cup. Place the tin into the preheated oven and bake for about 15 minutes (respect the recommended timing as they should not be overcooked). Turn the oven off and leave the tins inside so the muffins can cool for at least 20 minutes. Then, remove them from the tins and cover with plastic wrap and refrigerate. Serve them cold with sprinkled cinnamon on top. For garnishing, you can use a dab of sour cream with lemon zest or some fresh fruits like strawberries, blueberries, peach or apple.

Chocolate -Banana Grahams (71 calories and 13-gram carb per serving)

For one cracker serving you will need:

- 1 Graham cracker

- 1 teaspoon of Nutella nut spread

- Half a teaspoon of coconut sprinkles

Directions:

The directions are quite simple with this very easy snack. Spread the Nutella on top of the cracker, then place a slice of banana, sprinkle with some coconut, and voila!

Sugar-Free Fudge (147 cal., 5-gram carbs per serving)

For 16 servings you will need:

- 2-8 oz. packages of reduced fat cream cheese

- 2-1 oz. squares of unsweetened chocolate melted and cooled

- Some sugar substitute (which should be equal to 1 cup of sugar)

- 1 teaspoon of vanilla

- 1/2 cup of chopped pecan nuts

Directions:

In a small bowl, beat the cream cheese with the chocolate, sweetener and vanilla until smooth. Stir in the pecans, then put the mixture into an 8-inch square pan lined with foil. Cover the mixture and refrigerate overnight. Cut into 16 squares and serve chilled.

Evening Snacks

Back in the days, it was important for people who would have their pre-dinner insulin doses to snack before bedtime, so that they can avoid hypoglycemia (a dangerous condition where your blood sugar level crashes considerably).

Today, medical technology has improved and so did the insulin shots. There are now fewer risks to have these sorts of problems. But there is still a minority of people who experience this discomfort at night. So, for you, I've put up a list of light evening snacks that will help you go to bed without the risk of falling ill or gaining weight.

Here's a list of healthy snacks that you can eat before bedtime:

- You can go for a cup of strawberries (250 ml) with about ½ a cup of skimmed milk.

- You can also have some low fat cheese (about an ounce) with 4 whole grain crackers.

- Another option would be to simply have a cup of delicious blueberries.

- For those who love their dairies, 175 ml of sugar-free low-fat plain yogurt would do to fill you up before bedtime.

- You can also indulge in some air-popped popcorn (about 3 cups) if you want to.

All of these snacks are naturally sweet and fat-free, so you will not only maintain your insulin levels but maintain a healthy weight, as well.

Chapter 4: The Best Recipes for Lunch

Lunch is the best time for diabetics to really enjoy their food. You will find some very simple recipes that will help you have an idea of what a low fat, low carb tasty meal should really look like.

Entrées:

Barley and Black Bean Salad (349 cal., 53.2-gram carb per serving)

For 4 servings you will need:

- 1 cup of uncooked quick-cooking pearl barley
- 1 can of black beans (15oz), rinsed and drained
- Halved cherry tomatoes
- 1/2 cup of finely chopped green bell pepper
- 1/2 cup of Monterey Jack cheese with jalapeño peppers, cut into 1/4-inch cubes
- 1/3 cup of lemon juice
- 2 tablespoons of olive oil
- 1 teaspoon of salt
- 3/4 cup of fresh cilantro leaves
- 1/8 teaspoon of ground red pepper

Directions:

Begin by cooking your barley by simply following the package directions but, without adding salt. Then, drain the barley in a colander, and rinse with cold water until completely cooled. Next, combine the black beans, the remaining 6 ingredients, the cilantro and red pepper in a medium bowl. Add the barley to the black bean mixture and toss gently.

Veggie Tostadas (215 cal., 38.7gram carbs per serving)

For 4 servings you will need:

- Some cooking spray
- 2 cups of sliced mushrooms
- 2 small sliced zucchini
- 1 large chopped red bell pepper

Directions:

Begin your preparation with Placing a medium nonstick pan coated with cooking spray over medium-high heat, until hot. Add the mushrooms, the zucchini, and the bell pepper to the pan. Sauté for 3 to 5 minutes or until the vegetables are tender. Spoon about 3/4 cup vegetable mixture over black bean mixture on each tostada. Top with lettuce, salsa, and cheese.

Main course meals:

Basil Scallops with Spinach Fettucine (375 cal., 36.9-gram carbs per serving)

For four servings you will need:

- 8 ounces of uncooked spinach fettuccine

- 1 1/2 pounds of sea scallops
- 3/4 teaspoon of freshly ground black pepper
- Cooking spray
- 2 tablespoons of extra virgin olive oil
- 1 tablespoon of Dijon mustard
- 1 tablespoon of chopped fresh basil
- 1/4 teaspoon of salt
- 3/4 of a cup of dry white wine (or low-sodium chicken broth)
- 1/3 cup of finely chopped green onion
- 3 tablespoons of chopped fresh parsley

Directions:

First, cook the pasta following the package directions without the salt and fat. Drain when done. Rinse the scallops, and pat them dry with a paper towel. Then, sprinkle them with pepper. Place a large nonstick pan coated with cooking spray over medium-high heat until hot. Add half of the scallops; cook 3 minutes on each side. Remove the scallops from the pan and keep warm. Repeat the procedure with the remaining scallops. Combine the olive oil with the next 3 ingredients and set aside. Place the same pan over high heat until hot. Add the wine and green onions, and cook for 1 minute. Add the olive oil mixture; cook for 15 seconds. Add the scallops and the accumulated juices and cook for 15 seconds, stirring constantly. End the process by spooning the scallops and juices over the pasta. Sprinkle with parsley.

Snapper with Tomato Caper Topping (215 cal., 5.8-gram carb per serving)

For 4 servings you will need:

- 2 cups of halved grape tomatoes
- 2 tablespoons of drained capers
- 2 tablespoons of fresh lemon juice
- 2 teaspoons of olive oil
- 1 1/2 teaspoons dried of fresh basil
- 1/4 teaspoon of salt
- 1/8 teaspoon of crushed red pepper
- 4 grouper fillets (about 3/4 inch thick)
- Cooking spray
- 1 teaspoon of paprika
- 2 tablespoons of chopped fresh parsley
- 1 lemon, cut into 4 wedges

Directions:

Preheat the oven to 450°. Combine the first 6 ingredients and crushed red pepper; then, set aside. Place your snapper on a broiler pan lined with aluminum foil; coat the foil with cooking spray. Sprinkle the snapper with paprika and coat with cooking spray. Bake at 450° for 10 minutes. Then, top the snapper with your tomato mixture. Bake for 5 minutes. Sprinkle with parsley, and serve with lemon wedges.

Veggie Sausage-Cheddar Frittata (184 cal. and 10.4-gram Carbs per serving)

For 4 servings you will need:

- Some cooking spray
- A chopped green bell pepper
- 1 package of pre-sliced mushrooms (8oz)
- 4 frozen vegetable protein sausage patties, thawed and crumbled
- 1/8 teaspoon of salt
- 1/8 teaspoon of freshly ground black pepper
- 1 cup of egg substitute
- 1/4 cup of fat-free half-and-half
- 1/2 cup of shredded reduced-fat sharp Cheddar cheese (2oz)

Directions:

Preheat your broiler. Then, place a 12-inch ovenproof nonstick pan over medium-high heat. Coat your pan with some cooking spray. Add your chopped bell pepper and mushrooms and sauté for 3 minutes. Add the sausage, salt, and pepper and reduce the heat to medium-low. Cook for 1 minute. Combine the egg substitute and half-and-half and carefully pour over sausage mixture. Cover and cook for 6 minutes. The frittata should be slightly moist on top. Sprinkle with cheese and serve.

Desserts

Honey Grapefruit with bananas (122 cal., 31.3-gram carbs per serving)
For 3 servings you will need:

- A 24-ounce jar of refrigerated red grapefruit sections
- 1 sliced banana
- 1 tablespoon of fresh chopped mint
- 1 tablespoon of honey

Directions:

Drain the grapefruit sections and keep 1/4 cup of the juice. In a medium bowl, combine the grapefruit sections, the juice, and remaining ingredients. Toss gently to coat. This dish should be served immediately or covered and refrigerated for later.

Cantaloupe sherbet (93 cal., 18.9-gram carb per serving)
For 5 servings you will need:

- 1 large ripe cantaloupe, peeled and finely chopped
- 1/3 cup calorie-free sweetener
- 2 tablespoons of lemon juice
- 2 teaspoons of unflavored gelatin
- 1/4 cup of cold water

- 1 carton of vanilla fat-free yogurt sweetened with aspartame (8oz)
- Cantaloupe wedges

Directions:

Begin by combining the cantaloupe, the sweetener and lemon juice in a blender and mix until smooth. Transfer the mixture to a medium bowl. Sprinkle the gelatin over cold water in a small saucepan and let it stand for one minute. Then, cook over low heat, stirring until the gelatin has dissolved for about 4 minutes. Add to the cantaloupe mixture while stirring. Add yogurt and stir until smooth. Pour the mixture into an 8-inch square pan and freeze until it's almost firm. Transfer the mixture to a large bowl; beat with a mixer at high speed until it becomes fluffy. Spoon the mixture back into the pan and freeze again until firm.

Scoop your sherbet into 5 individual serving dishes to serve. Finish by garnishing each serving with a cantaloupe wedge. Enjoy!

Chapter 5: Dinner Is Served!

As you know it already, the perfect night time meal shouldn't be too heavy. The rule applies to diabetics too, except that they can be allowed to have a night time snack, every now and then.

In this chapter, you will find great delicious meals that are just under 200 calories, but will still fill you up for the night. And instead of having some dessert, you can simply have an apple or a 100% fruit juice, fruit salad, that are both low in carbs and very nutritious.

Dinner Recipe Number One: Chicken Skewers with Peach Salsa (171 cal., 9-gram carb per serving)

You will need:

- 3 tablespoons of rice vinegar

- 1 tablespoon of reduced-sodium soy sauce

- 1 teaspoon of packed brown sugar or brown sugar substitute

- 1 teaspoon of grated fresh ginger

- 8 ounces of skinless, boneless chicken breast halves, cut lengthwise into 1-inch strips

- 1/2 of a medium peach, pitted and chopped

- 2 tablespoons of chopped red sweet pepper

- 2 teaspoons of finely chopped red onion

- 2 teaspoons of snipped fresh cilantro

- 1/2 teaspoon of lime juice

- 1/4 teaspoon of finely chopped, seeded fresh jalapeno chile pepper

Directions:

Use a large resealable plastic bag that you will set in a deep bowl to combine the rice vinegar, soy sauce, brown sugar, and ginger. Next, add the chicken strips. Seal the bag and turn to coat chicken. Let it marinate in the refrigerator for 2 to 4 hours, turning the bag occasionally. Drain the chicken by discarding the marinade. Thread the chicken onto two 10- to 12-inch-long skewers.

Grill the skewers on the rack of an uncovered grill directly over medium coals for 5 to 7 minutes, turning occasionally to brown it evenly. If you are using a gas grill, preheat your grill. Reduce the heat to medium and place the chicken skewers on grill rack over heat.

For the peach salsa use a small bowl to combine your peach, sweet pepper, onion, cilantro, lime juice, and jalapeno pepper.

Serve the chicken skewers with peach salsa. Bon appetite!

Dinner Recipe Number Two: Green Beans with Cilantro (50 cal., 7-gram carbs per serving).

For 2 servings you will need:

- 6 ounces of fresh trimmed green beans

- 1 garlic clove, minced

- 1 teaspoon of olive oil

- 1/8 teaspoon of salt

- 1/8 teaspoon of ground black pepper

- 1 tablespoon of snipped fresh cilantro

Directions:

First, place a steamer basket in a large saucepan with a tight-fitting lid. Add some water to just below the basket. Then, bring your water to boiling over medium-high heat. Place the beans in the steamer basket. Cover and steam for 8 to 10 minutes (the beans should be crisp-tender). In a large nonstick pan, cook the garlic in hot oil over medium heat for 15 seconds. Stir constantly. Add the beans, salt, and pepper. Cook for 3 more minutes, tossing occasionally. Sprinkle with cilantro and enjoy.

Dinner Recipe Number Three: Seared Scallops with Mint Pesto (189 cal., 7-gram carbs per serving)

For 2 servings you will need:

- 1/3 cup of lightly packed fresh mint

- 1/4 cup of lightly packed fresh flat-leaf parsley

- 2 tablespoons of toasted and chopped almonds

- 2 tablespoons of grated Parmesan cheese

- 2 tablespoons of water

- 1 tablespoon of lemon juice

- 2 minced garlic cloves

- 1/4 teaspoon of salt

- 1/4 teaspoon of ground black pepper

- 6 sea scallops (8 to 10 ounces in total)

- 1 teaspoon of olive oil

- 1 cup of fresh watercress (or spinach)

Directions:

For the pesto use a food processor to combine the mint, parsley, almonds, Parmesan cheese, the water, lemon juice, garlic, 1/8 teaspoon of the salt, and 1/8 teaspoon of the pepper. Cover and process until everything are nearly smooth, then set aside.

Rinse your scallops and pat dry with paper towels. Sprinkle your scallops with the remaining 1/8 teaspoon of salt and 1/8 teaspoon of pepper. In a large nonstick pan, heat some oil over medium-high heat. Add the scallops and cook for about 4 to 5 minutes. Turn once halfway through cooking.

To finish, serve the scallops and pesto over watercress.

Dinner Recipe Number Four: Southwestern Skirt Steak (196 cal., 2- gram carbs per serving)

For 2 servings you will need:

- 1/3 cup of orange juice

- 2 tablespoons of snipped fresh cilantro

- 2 tablespoons of lime juice

- 1 teaspoon of ground cumin

- 1/4 teaspoon of salt

- 1/4 teaspoon of ground black pepper

- 1 minced garlic clove

- 8 ounces of beef skirt steak (or flank steak)

Directions:

Use a large resealable plastic bag (set in a shallow baking dish) to combine the orange juice, the cilantro, lime juice, cumin, salt, pepper, and garlic. Trim the fat from the steak and discard it. Score both sides of the steak in a diamond pattern by making shallow diagonal cuts at 1-inch intervals. Add the steak to the orange juice mixture. Seal the bag and turn to coat the steak. Then, let marinate in the refrigerator for 1 to 4 hours, turning the bag occasionally. Drain the steak and discard the marinade.

For a charcoal grill, place your steak on the rack of an uncovered grill directly over medium coals. Grill until the desired doneness, turning once halfway through grilling. For skirt steak, allow 8 to 10 minutes. For flank steak, allow 10 to 12 minutes for medium-rare doneness (145 degrees F) or 12 to 14 minutes for medium doneness (160 degrees F). If you are using a gas grill, preheat the grill. Reduce the heat to medium. Place the steak on the grill rack over heat. Cover and grill as above.

To serve, thinly slice the steak across the grain, and Bon appetite!

Chapter 6: Your Beverages

Water (distilled or filtered) is the most recommended drink for people with diabetes. Hopefully, they can still enjoy any other beverages as long as they are low in sugar but rich in nutritional value (that's one of the advantages of being diabetic). Let's now discover some of the non-alcoholic options that you can even make at home.

Your Hot Beverages

Hot Chocolate Milk (70 cal., 16-grams carbs per serving)

Mix together 1% milk and 3 teaspoons of cocoa powder and 2 tablespoons of zero calories of a sweetener of your choice. Warm it up for 1 and a half seconds, and enjoy while warm.

Chai Latte (less than 1 gram of carbs)

Put 1 or 2 of chai tea bags in a cup of unsweetened almond milk and spice it up with some cinnamon and black pepper to add some extra flavor to it.

Café Mocha (less than 60 cal. and 10-gram carbs per serving)

Mix up 1 cup of brewed coffee with a tablespoon of cocoa powder. Then, add 2 tablespoons of low-fat milk and a little bit of your zero-calorie sugar substitute.

Cold Beverages

Orange Juice (15 cal., 3 grams of carbs per serving)

Buy a flavored light fruit juice from now on, or simply make your own (unsweetened version at home). You simply can put peeled oranges in your grinder to make you a fresh cup in the morning.

Lemonade (0 cal., 0 grams of carbs per serving)

Mix some fresh squeezed lemons with some water. Add your zero calorie sweetener and some ice and voila!

A fruit smoothie (less than 90 cal. and 20 grams carbs per serving)

Blend half a cup of blueberries with the same amounts of bananas and strawberries (half a cup each) blend the whole with some ice and drink immediately to savor this refreshing drink.

You can also drink a cup of regular coffee or any diet sodas available out there. Just make sure you avoid sugary drinks as they contain too much sugar with just one serving (it's 150 calories and 40 grams of carbs for 12 ounces of a regular can of soda).

Conclusion

Thank you again for downloading this book!

I hope this book was able to help you have an idea of what cooking should really be for people with diabetes.

The next step is to learn more about the food that is right for you by setting up a chart. Don't forget to always have a list of your "always necessary items" every time you go out grocery shopping.

As a diabetic who wants to have better options when it comes to eating, you should:

- Consider your weight, age, gender, and lifestyle to know how much food you really need to eat, every day.

- Plan your meals ahead and see if you will need a midday or evening snack, especially when you are taking medication.

- Know your "carbs" and calorie counts, every time you pick a meal.

- Remember to read the label of the food you buy to make sure if what you are buying is diabetic safe.

- Don't be afraid to ask the staff at your job's cafeteria for advice or information on the food served there, or available menus for diabetics.

- Don't be afraid to be curious about your own meal options and enjoy good food. Don't let your disease cut you out from some life pleasures.

Truly enjoy your meals, from now on!

Special Bonus Only For My Readers

If you liked this book and would like to get my new books FREE on release, don't forget to get into my V.I.P. list where you will get first hand on my new personal development books. Once the V.I.P. group is filled up, I will no longer be accepting more members.

GET INTO THE EXCLUSIVE GROUP HERE

Or go to http://tokkul.com/personal-development

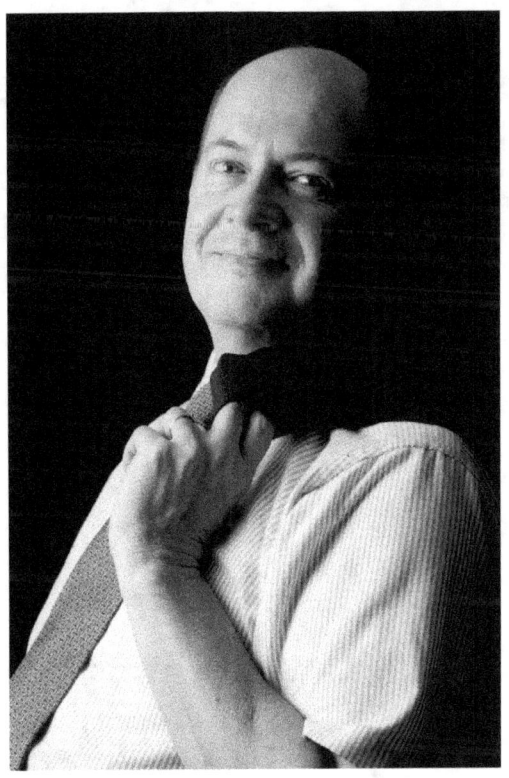

Thank you again for downloading this book!

If you enjoyed this book, then I'd like to ask you for a favor, would you be kind enough to leave a review for this book on Amazon? It'd be greatly appreciated!

Thank you and good luck!

Stevie Anderson

www.ingramcontent.com/pod-product-compliance
Lightning Source LLC
Chambersburg PA
CBHW071142280526
45787CB00003B/1379